Souleymane MAÏGA

STUDY OF THE DISPENSING OF ANTI-CANCER DRUGS

Souleymane MAÏGA

STUDY OF THE DISPENSING OF ANTI-CANCER DRUGS

Study of the dispensing of anticancer drugs in the private pharmacy M'PEWO, Bamako-Mali

ScienciaScripts

Imprint
Any brand names and product names mentioned in this book are subject to trademark, brand or patent protection and are trademarks or registered trademarks of their respective holders. The use of brand names, product names, common names, trade names, product descriptions etc. even without a particular marking in this work is in no way to be construed to mean that such names may be regarded as unrestricted in respect of trademark and brand protection legislation and could thus be used by anyone.

Cover image: www.ingimage.com

This book is a translation from the original published under ISBN 978-620-6-72133-8.

Publisher:
Sciencia Scripts
is a trademark of
Dodo Books Indian Ocean Ltd. and OmniScriptum S.R.L publishing group

120 High Road, East Finchley, London, N2 9ED, United Kingdom
Str. Armeneasca 28/1, office 1, Chisinau MD-2012, Republic of Moldova, Europe
Printed at: see last page
ISBN: 978-620-8-31141-4

DEDICATION

I dedicate this work

To my dear grandfather, the late Mamadou TRAORE

You have always been an example to me of a respectful, honest and meticulous father, and I want to honour the man you were. Thanks to you Baba I have learnt the meaning of work and responsibility. I'd like to thank you for your love, your generosity, your understanding... Your support has been a beacon throughout my career. This modest work is the fruit of all the sacrifices you made for my education and training. I implore the Almighty to grant you his immense paradise, amen.

To my dear grandmother, the late Nassé DIARRA

So many sentences, no matter how expressive, could never show the degree of love and affection I feel for you. You showered me with your tenderness and affection throughout my life, right up to your last breath. You never ceased to support and encourage me throughout the years of your life. On this memorable day, for me as well as for you, receive this work as a sign of my deep gratitude and my profound esteem. May the Almighty grant you his immense paradise, amen.

To my father Ibrahim MAIGA

Thank you for everything, Father, for your encouragement and support. Despite the distance between us I can never thank you enough, but I know that today you would be very proud of me. May the Almighty give you long life in health and prosperity.

To my dear mother Hawa TRAORE

There are no words that can adequately express my love and attachment to you. Giving me life is the greatest gift you have ever given me. An affectionate woman, a generous woman, a hard-working woman, a patient woman, a courageous woman, a virtuous woman, these are the qualities that make you an admirable person. Everything I am today I owe to you. I can't find the words to express my gratitude for all the sacrifices you make every day for my sister and me. May the Almighty give you health, happiness and long life so that I can fulfil you in my turn.

To My Uncle Boubacar TRAORE

THANKS

I'll never find enough words to express my gratitude. You have always put our studies above everything else. Through our education, you are and always will be an exemplary role model for us. While praying to God to grant you good health and a long life, I dedicate this work to you, which represents the culmination of the support and encouragement you have given me throughout my schooling, and I hope that you will always be proud of me. I thank you most sincerely for your advice, your encouragement, your sense of a job well done and above all for accepting me as your own son. May the good GOD grant you the best and guide you unceasingly in righteousness.

To my aunt Habibatou TRAORE

A generous woman, a fighter, courageous and responsible. Godmother to all the children in the Salifoubougou family, your generosity has been and always will be a source of motivation for me. On behalf of the whole family, thank you and thank you again, Tante Habi. May the good Lord grant you a very long life of happiness, health and kindness.

To my Uncles and Aunts Salif TRAORE, Hamidou TRAORE, the late Issouf TRAORE, the late Ibrahim TRAORE, the late Mamoutou TRAORE, Mamadou TRAORE, Maimouna TRAORE, Fanta TRAORE, Bintou TRAORE, Sitan TRAORE, Sira TRAORE and collecgues de services, Fily Christine KEITA, Djeneba BAMBERA, Setou DIALLO, Mah SYLLA, Sitan DIARRA, Awa FOFANA Your blessings, advice and encouragement have been a great support to me along the way. THANK YOU!

To my fiancée Hawa DOUMBIA

You've been more than a wife to me, given your love, your courage, your support and the difficulties you've put up with. May this thesis be the starting point for a better future. Amen to that!

To my sister Fanta COUMARE and all my Cousins and Cousines

Thank you all for your blessings, your support, your encouragement and above all your love and consideration for me. May the Almighty unite us and strengthen us.

To all the members of the Salifoubougou family

What can I say? How do I express what I'm feeling? Where do I find the right words to thank you? Host family, hospitality, I can't thank you enough for everything you've done for me. the *support I have received from you. This is the moment to express my gratitude. I hope that you will find in this work, the testimony of my most sincere and affectionate feelings. May Allah protect you, give you good health and help you to fulfil your most cherished wishes. Thank you for your kindness!*

ACKNOWLEDGEMENTS

To Allah, the Almighty, the Creator and the Most Merciful, we give You thanks by saying Alhamdoulilah !!! Thank You for giving me the health, the ability to think, to perform and to write, to make my dream come true.To the Prophet: May God bestow His blessing and salvation on Our Prophet Muhammad, his family, his companions and all those who follow in their footsteps until the Day of Resurrection.

To my beautiful country, Mali

You enabled me to take my first steps towards learning. You gave me immeasurable knowledge; I am deeply grateful to my beloved country.

To all my teachers, from primary to secondary level, and to all the teaching staff of the Faculty of Pharmacy (FAPH)

Your high-quality courses, your teaching techniques and your encouragement have spurred us on. to achieve this excellence. Thank you for everything you have done for our training.

To my very dear primary school teacher Aminata TRAORE and my very dear secondary school teachers Mr BERTHE and Mr Thomas BOFFI

I can never thank you enough, you have been more than just teachers to me, you have supported, encouraged and helped me at every stage of my school life. You have placed your hopes and ambitions in me, the extent of which I am still unaware, and this has always enabled me to move forward safely, even in difficult times. May GOD reward you for all your good deeds and grant you a long and healthy life of happiness. Thank you very much!

To Professor Oumar SANGHO

You have been more than a guide, your professionalism will certainly inspire me in my professional life. In this work you will find the fulfilment of your vocation.

To my masters Doctor Moussa Modibo DIARRA and Doctor Abou SOGODOGO

No words or expressions would suffice to thank you and express my feelings of respect, because your profession will never be remunerated at its fair value. Thank you for your guidance. May God grant you a long life full of health, happiness and success.

To the staff and other PhD students of the Health Teaching and Research Department public Thank you for your cooperation and courtesy. Good luck to all of us. To Doctor Moussa Almamy COULIBALY, promoter of the M'PEWO Pharmacy

A pious, generous, hard-working and ambitious man, you welcomed me into your pharmacy like a son and gave me the opportunity to receive high-quality training. I can never thank you enough. May Allah protect you and grant you your wishes.

To the staff of Pharmacie M'PEWO

You taught me good pharmacy practice and you gave me all the help I needed to complete this work, all credit to you. May God keep us together and help me to be grateful to you.

To Manager Mohamed SIDIBE and his staff and the entire 15th class of the Numerus clausus Pr Saïbou MAIGA promotion

Thank you for the love, the fraternity, the solidarity and the long road we have travelled together. Good luck to you all in your future professional lives.

To my classmates Adama POUDIOUGO, Nouh BAMADIO, Dr Kalifa OUATTARA, Souleymane COULIBALY, Issa Tieko DIABATE, Dr Abdoulaye SARAMBOUNOU, Abdrahamane Salif KAMATE, Seydou SOUMAORO, Fatoumata Zahara BARRY, Dr Ibrahim B MAIGA, Dr Mohamed S Diarra, Amadou SAMASSEKOU, Dr Binta KRAMA, Boubacar SOW, Mamadou Fode DIEFAGA, Bakary DJIRE, Founè MANGARA, Ibrahim MBODJI, Youba TOGO, Mahamane TOURE, Yelly CISSE

We've been through some difficult times together. Thank you for your invaluable support. More than friends, you are brothers and sisters to me. May there be understanding between us forever.

To Dr Cheick Oumar KONE "Dr Hassala

You are my brother from another mother whom God has blessed me with. To all the times we spent together, to all our memories! Thank you for being there every step of the way. I'm honoured to have you in my life and I wish you all the happiness and success you deserve. As a tribute to our beautiful friendship and to the years to come. May our friendship be eternal, and may the special bond we have forged over the years be eternally unbreakable.

To Dr Fatoumata SIDIBE

Thank you for the quality of your teaching, your advice, your encouragement and especially your presence which I benefited from during this thesis, may Allah grant you a good career continuation. Amen!

To Mamadou Boye BA

Thank you for your help in preparing this thesis. Good luck and good courage for the the rest of your studies.

To Uncle IBE DIARRA

Thank you for everything Uncle, no words can express your generosity. May Allah give you a very long life in good health and may he grant you a good professional career. Amen!

To Doctor Abdouramane BA, Doctor Seydou Doumbia, Bréhima DEMBELE, Doctor Cheick Oumar DIARRA, Doctor Ibrahim SIDIBE, Doctor Modibo TRAORE, Doctor Fatoumata TOURE, Arouna KONATE, Seydou DEMBELE, Andre KOUNDOUNOU and to my pharmacy training colleagues M'PEWO Bagnini DIALLO, Saïdou Gouro DIALL, Mohamed Z SANOGO, Abdoulaye CAMARA, Jacques KOUMEDJINA.

Thank you for the fraternity, the complicity and your commitment in drawing up this document. May God grant us many good moments together.

To my brothers and childhood accomplices OG Loup, Guepa Bling, Sora F16, Med Moh King, Nescofa, ZP kegno, Brom Chee, Flaga, Toczer CFA, Alove Chee, Baye Chee, Ramichka, N

I don't have the words to describe the feeling that unites us, but one thing's for sure, wherever we are, whatever the conditions, you'll always be my friends, you'll always be my brothers and sisters. To all the members of Cité OUA, especially to KBG members Abass KONATE, Souleymane Berthé, Souleymane DIAKITE, Cedric BAKANBOU, Abdoulaye CAMARA, Alice DOUGNON, Assetou DIARRA (Double Seven), Aïchatou DEMBELE, Issa SIDIBE, Daouda BAGAYOKO, BEN, TEFOUROU, Le grand SORIBA, Mamadou SANGARE, Makan, MAREGA, Nouhoum COULIBALY, Oumar Fakourou, Oumou NIKLA, Yaya SISSOKO, Laya DJIBO, PriscaDani, Dr Tatiana, Ulrich, Rokia, Nana Kadia,

Thank you for your invaluable support. More than friends, you are brothers and sisters to me. ***To all those whom I have not mentioned: who are dear to me, the error is human and this is far from being a deliberate intention on my part, but it in no way detracts from the fact that I hold you in my heart. Please accept my apologies.***

TRIBUTES TO THE MEMBERS OF THE JURY

Professor Hamadoun SANGHO

- ***Professor Full of Health Public Health à the Faculty of Medicine and Odontostomatology (FMOS);***
- ***Head of the Department of Teaching and Research (DER) in Public Health at the Faculty of Medicine and Odontostomatology;***
- ***Former Director General Manager of the former of Research, Study and de Documentation pour la Survie de l'enfant (CREDOS) ;***
- ***Knight of the National Order of Mali.***

Dear Master,

You do us a great honour by agreeing to chair this jury. Your admirable scientific, social and moral qualities and your simplicity make you a Master respected by all, and also testify to the importance you attach to training. Dear Master, allow us to express our humble and profound gratitude. May the Almighty Allah grant you a long life.

TO OUR MASTER AND JUDGE

Professor Yeya dit Sadio SARRO

- ***Lecturer in Epidemiology at the Faculty of Pharmacy (FAPH);***
- ***Epidemiologist at the Centre de Recherche et de Lutte Contre la Drépanocytose ;***
- ***Senior researcher at the University Clinical Research Center (UCRC).***

Dear Master,

We were not surprised that you agreed to sit on this jury, given your love of a job well done and your availability for student training. Your modesty, scientific rigour and human qualities make you an admired and respected teacher. It is an honour for us to have you as a member and judge, may God grant you longevity, health and happiness.

TO OUR MASTER AND JUDGE

Dr Moussa Almamy COULIBALY

- ***Doctor of Pharmacy ;***
- ***Promoter of the M'PEWO pharmacy;***
- ***Member of the SYNAPPO national bureau since 1996;***
- ***Vice-Chairman of SYNAPPO ;***
- ***Founding member of the African International Pharmaceutical Forum;***
- ***Director of Laborex Mali since 2012.***

Dear Master,

Despite your many activities, you have done us the honour of agreeing to correct and judge this work with rigour and objectivity. Your human and intellectual qualities, your simplicity and your scientific qualities make you an example to follow. Please accept our deepest gratitude and sincere thanks.

TO OUR MASTER AND CO-THESIS DIRECTOR Pr Issa COULIBALY

- ***Lecturer in Management at the FMOS and the FAPH;***
- ***Head of the FAPH examinations and competitions department ;***
- ***Master's degree in management of healthcare establishments;***
- ***Ph D in Management /UCAD Senegal ;***
- ***President of the Koulikoro Order of Pharmacists ;***
- ***Practising pharmacist at the Pr BSS University Hospital in Kati.***

Dear Master,

Your broad scientific knowledge and intellectual honesty have won our admiration. We are very proud and honoured to be counted among your disciples. Dear Master, it is a great pleasure to express to you here, solemnly, our deep gratitude and our sincere thanks.

TO OUR MASTER AND THESIS DIRECTOR

Professor Oumar SANGHO

- ***Associate Professor of Epidemiology ;***
- ***PhD in Epidemiology;***
- ***EPIVAC Inter-University Diploma (DIU) ;***
- ***Health Promotion Certificate ;***
- ***Lecturer and researcher at the Department of Teaching and Research in Public Health and Specialities (DERSP) / FMOS / USTTB ;***
- ***Former Chief Medical Officer of the Niono Health District.***

Dear Master

We are very grateful to you for the welcome and guidance we received throughout our stay in the Department of Teaching and Research in Public Health and Specialties. Your human and intellectual qualities, your generosity, your friendliness, your availability to our many requests and your collaboration were of particular interest. Rest assured that your advice and teaching have not been in vain and that we are very proud to be counted among your students.

TABLE OF CONTENTS

INTRODUCTION

Cancer is a disease characterised by the uncontrolled proliferation of cells, linked to an escape from the regulatory mechanisms that ensure the harmonious development of our body and the coexistence between normal cells (1). Cancer is one of the leading causes of morbidity and mortality in the world (2), and the number of new cases of cancer worldwide is expected to rise from 14 million in 2012 to almost 22 million in 2030 (2). According to the World Health Organisation (WHO), there are around 1.1 million new cases of cancer in Africa every year, and up to 700,000 deaths from the disease (3). Cancer is the cause of almost 10 million deaths by 2020, and is responsible for one in six deaths worldwide (4). Around 70% of these deaths occur in low- and middle-income countries (4).According to Globocan, 72.15% of the 14,185 new cases of cancer in Mali in 2020 were fatal (5). A retrospective study revealed that 31.8% of the 924 cases of cancer had not received appropriate treatment (4).Breast cancer, along with cervical, prostate, liver and colorectal cancer, accounts for almost half of all new cases of cancer reported on the continent each year (3).urbanisation, the incidence of infectious diseases such as AIDS, the lack of of health workers trained in cancer treatment, and a lack of dedicated facilities and equipment (6). The WHO stresses that "poverty" is a determining factor in the prevalence of cancer (7). African patients are only diagnosed at an advanced stage (stage 2 or 3) of the disease (7). Health professionals are alarmed and fear that cancer will "soon become the leading cause of death in Africa" (6). Africa suffers from unequal access to healthcare and a lack of prevention (7).Chemotherapy, hormone therapy, surgery and radiotherapy are the mainstays of cancer treatment (7). Cancer treatment is a real challenge in developing countries, particularly Mali (7). Late diagnosis, the non-availability of certain therapeutic means and anti-cancer drugs and the high cost of treatment are reasons that may explain the lack of access to these therapies. (8). According to a study carried out at the hospital pharmacy of the CHU du Point G in 2022, the average percentage of anticancer drugs available was 63.64%, hindering the continuity of free care and prolonging waiting times for chemotherapy (4). The M'PEWO pharmacy is one of the largest pharmacies in Mali and a reference in terms of dispensing anti-cancer products. Given the scarcity of studies on anti-cancer drugs in private pharmacies, we felt it was important to carry out this study in the said pharmacy.

OBJECTIVES

2.1. General objective :

Study the dispensing of anti-cancer drugs in the M'PEWO private pharmacy from August 2023 to July 2024.

2.2. Specific objectives :

- Determine the socio-demographic characteristics of patients undergoing anti-cancer treatment;
- Identify the type of cancer or diseased organ in patients;
- Identify the regulatory characteristics of prescriptions;
- To determine the availability of anti-cancer molecules used in the management of cancer requested from the M'PEWO pharmacy;
- Identify the anti-cancer molecules used in cancer treatment requested from the M'PEWO pharmacy;
- Determine the average price of anticancer drugs charged at the M'PEWO pharmacy.

GENERAL

3.1. CANCER

3.1.1.Definition (1):

Cancer is a disease caused by an initially normal cell whose programme goes awry and transforms it. It multiplies and produces abnormal cells that proliferate in an uncontrolled and excessive manner. By multiplying in an uncontrolled way and modifying their environment, cancer cells give rise to increasingly large tumours that develop by invading and then destroying the areas around them (organs). Cancer cells can also spread away from an organ to form a new tumour (metastasis), or circulate in free form. In medicine, the term tumour (from the Latin tumere, to swell) refers to an increase in the volume of a tissue, without specifying the cause. It is a new formation of body tissue (neoplasia) that occurs as a result of a disturbance in cell growth, either benign or malignant (when it is a malignant tumour, it is called cancer) (9).

3.1.2.Types of cancer(10)

The different types of cancer are determined by their histology, in other words the nature of the tissue in which they develop. A distinction is made between :

- Carcinomas: the cancerous cells appear in an epithelium, i.e. a tissue covering the internal surfaces (organ lining tissue) or external surfaces (epidermis, for example). This family includes adenocarcinomas, which develop from the epithelium of glands such as the breast and prostate.
- Sarcomas: the cancerous cells appear in a "support" tissue such as bone, fat or muscle. These are called osteosarcomas (bone sarcomas), liposarcomas (fatty tissue sarcomas) and rhabdomyosarcomas (striated muscle sarcomas).
- Haematopoietic or haematological cancers: cancerous cells appear in the bone marrow, which produces blood cells (red and white blood cells and platelets) and their precursors. They may also appear in other lymphoid organs (thymus, lymph nodes, etc.), spleen, tonsils, etc.). There are three families of haematological cancers: leukaemia, myeloma and lymphoma.

3.1.3.Classification and staging of cancers (10) :

Cancer develops differently depending on whether it is a solid tumour (carcinoma or sarcoma) or a haematopoietic cancer. At the time of diagnosis, as well as identifying the type of cancer, doctors define the degree of spread of the disease (based on the extent and volume of the tumour), i.e. its stage. To do this, they use classification systems.

- Classification of solid tumours :

To determine the stage of the cancer, doctors most often use an international classification system called TNM (Tumor, Node, Mestastasis), based on :

• The size of the tumour (T) ;

• Whether or not the lymph nodes are affected by cancer cells (N, from the English Node meaning lymph node);

• The presence or absence of metastases in other parts of the body (M).

There are 5 different stages, numbered from 0 to IV. Staging varies according to the type of cancer. Please note: There are also other classification systems for solid tumours, such as the FIGO classification for ovarian and cervical cancer, for example. It distinguishes five stages:

• Stage 0 corresponds to an in situ tumour;

• Stage 1 corresponds to a single, small tumour;

• Stage 2 corresponds to a larger local volume;

• Stage 3 corresponds to invasion of lymph nodes or neighbouring tissues;

• Stage 4 corresponds to a more extensive spread in the body in the form of metastases.

- Classification of haematopoietic cancers :

For haematopoietic cancers, each type of cancer has its own classification. For example, the Durie-Salmon classification is used for multiple myeloma. It determines 2 stages, A and B, on the basis of measurements of certain elements in the blood and X-rays of the skeleton.

3.1.4.Mechanism of carcinogenesis (11) :

Malignant transformation is the complex process by which cancerous cells develop from healthy cells. It involves several stages:

• Initiation: a change in the genetic material of a cell (mutation) prepares it to become malignant. A change in the cell's genetic material can occur spontaneously through a random event or genetic mutation, or be caused by external exposure to a substance that causes cancer (carcinogen).

• Promotion: The agents responsible, known as promoters, can be substances found in the external environment or certain drugs such as sex hormones (for example, testosterone taken to stimulate libido and sexual energy in older men). Unlike carcinogens, promoters are not in themselves the direct cause of cancer. However, they do enable the cell that has undergone initiation to become cancerous. However, promotion has no effect on non-initiated cells. Some carcinogens are powerful enough not to need promoters to induce cancer. For example, ionising radiation

• Spread: A cancer can develop (invade) directly in the surrounding tissue or spread to adjacent or distant tissues or organs. The disease can also spread through the lymphatic system, which is typical in the case of carcinomas. Only later does it spread to distant sites. The tumour can also spread through the bloodstream. This type of spread is typical of sarcomas.

3.1.5.History (7):

It was Hippocrates (460-377 BC), the father of Greek medicine, who gave his name to the disease: the word "cancer" comes from the Greek Latin "Karkinos" meaning "crab".

"This is the origin of the term "carcinoma" (another name for cancer). Hippocrates relied on the "theory of humours", a theory that prevailed until the middle of the 17ème century. This theory explained that most diseases, and cancers in particular, were caused by an imbalance between the four substances in the body: lymph (or phlegm), blood, the yellow bile produced by the liver and black bile.

3.1.6.Epidemiology (12):

Cancer is one of the leading causes of death in the world, accounting for almost 10 million deaths in 2020, or nearly one in six deaths. Every year, around 400,000 children develop cancer. The most common cancers in 2020 (in terms of new cases) were :

• Breast (2.26 million cases) ;

• Lung (2.21 million cases; 1.80 million deaths) ;

• Colon and rectum (1.93 million cases; 916,000 deaths) ;

• Prostate (1.41 million cases) ;

• Skin (other than melanoma) (1.20 million cases); and

• Stomach (1.09 million cases; 769,000 deaths).

Although the incidence of cancer is lower in Africa today than in the rest of the world, cancer

mortality is proportionately higher in Africa than elsewhere in the world, with an estimated 850,000 new cases and 590,000 deaths in 2012, 1
400,000 new cases and 1,050,000 deaths expected by 2030 (if no action is taken). Mali recorded 72.15% of deaths from 14,185 new cases of cancer in 2020 according to Globocan (5). According to Globocan, the number of new cancer cases is expected to rise from 14,200 in 2020 to 28,300 in 2040 (13). In 2019, 1,545 cases of cancer were recorded in the Bamako health district alone, according to the National Cancer Registry (14).

Cancer is treated in three public hospitals (Hôpital du Mali, CHU Gabriel Touré and CHU Point G). Only Mali Hospital has a radiotherapy department. The Point G and Gabriel Toure hospitals have seen a large number of cancer cases, with 41.4% and 25.9% respectively according to a retrospective study, which also highlights that in 2020 the majority of patients were female (59%, 1,4858 patients) (7).

3.1.7.Risk factors (10)

Cancer is never the result of a single cause. It takes a combination of factors, all of which are likely to interact, for the disease to develop. A number of these factors, both external and internal, have been identified.

- External factors :

They are linked to the environment (radiation, viruses, industrial products, etc.) or to lifestyle (smoking, alcohol, diet, etc.). There is evidence that repeated attacks on the DNA of cells by certain chemicals, such as tobacco, or by radiation (nuclear or solar) encourage the development of cancer cells. Viruses and bacteria can also be the cause of certain cancers, such as cervical cancer linked to the human papillomavirus, liver cancer linked to the hepatitis B virus, and stomach cancer linked to the Helicobacter pylori bacterium.

- Internal factors: These include age and heredity.

Ageing plays a fundamental role. Although cancers can appear at any age, they are much more common after the age of 60. This is due to the accumulation of external aggressions to which the cells are subjected and, probably, to the reduced efficiency of DNA repair mechanisms in older people.

Heredity can also play a role. Some people are more likely to develop cancer than others because, at birth, they already carry mutations in one or more of their genes, mutations inherited from their parents and present in all their cells.

➤ Genetic predisposition to cancer :

The mutation that occurs during cell division affects the DNA of a germline cell, in other words a cell involved in reproduction and fertilisation (ova and spermatozoa). This means that the mutation can be passed on to offspring. If this is the case, the mutation is present in all the cells of the offspring's body. When this type of mutation is implicated in a cancer, we speak of a hereditary form or a genetic predisposition to cancer.

3.2. CHEMOTHERAPY

3.2.1.Definition (15):

Chemotherapy is a treatment involving the administration of drugs that act on cancer cells, either by destroying them or by preventing them from multiplying. These drugs are not selective or targeted and act on other healthy cells in the body, particularly cells that multiply rapidly (bone marrow, hair, skin, etc.), which explains the side effects of chemotherapy. The aim of chemotherapy is to disrupt the processes essential to the multiplication of tumour cells.

3.2.2.History (7) :

Paul Ehrlich, winner of the Nobel Prize for Medicine in 1908, the birth of chemotherapy (not primarily to combat cancer, as we might think, but syphilis, which was all the rage at the dawn of the twentieth century). During the Second World War, American soldiers suffered the full force of the enemy's use of nitrogen mustard gas. They developed worrying symptoms, with an abnormal and significant drop in white blood cells. Two eminent pharmacologists from Yale University, Alfred Gilman and Louis Goodman, commissioned by the US Ministry of Defence, came up with the ingenious idea of using mustard agents to try to stem the inevitable, uncontrolled proliferation of white blood cells inherent in leukaemia. Tests on mice proved conclusive. In humans, a gas derived from mustard was injected intravenously to successfully treat non-Hodkignian lymphoma in 1946. However, the bone marrow failed and the mustard gas revealed its limitations, with the death of the patient in 1948. Improvements were more necessary than ever.

The first real anti-cancer chemotherapy was developed by Sidney Farber, a pathologist at Harvard University. He focused on folic acid (a vitamin that plays a key role in DNA metabolism). Surrounded by a circle of experts, he produced folate analogues, negating folic acid and, at the same time, the exponential growth of easily-divisible leukaemia cells. This led to the previously unthinkable: remission in children suffering from acute lymphoblastic leukaemia (one of the two forms of blood cancer that affects lymphocytes, whereas myeloid leukaemia affects polynuclear white blood cells). The little patients even had the pleasure of regaining normal bone marrow, as if the disease had only been a bad dream. However, methotrexate (its most effective agent) has revealed its limitations, with a rare complete cure.

Chemotherapy is now used on a large scale, and many specialists around the world are researching or developing new anti-cancer molecules with a wide range of administration methods. Their ideal aim is to reduce the legion of so-called 'side' or 'undesirable' effects that are so annoying for patients. Combination treatment is a beneficial approach, and one that has been exploited since the mid-1960s. Precision, with the focus solely on cancerous areas, has been improved for greater "comfort" , This is known as targeted therapy. While chemotherapy may still seem frightening at first sight, it is also a source of immense hope, which has now won over a patient base that is calmer inside and more confident in the light of the progress that is being made.

3.2.3.Types of chemotherapy (7) :

- Curative chemotherapy

Chemotherapy is the major step (usually complementary to another step) that can lead to recovery. If it is not carried out correctly, it can be a waste of time and compromise patients' chances of recovery.

- Adjuvant and neoadjuvant chemotherapy

• Adjuvant chemotherapy :

In this situation, chemotherapy is used because we know that, statistically, patients have a better chance of surviving with chemotherapy. However, for a given patient, this is not necessarily true: the undesirable effects of chemotherapy may cancel out the expected positive effect of chemotherapy. It may be prescribed after the most essential procedure (surgery or radiotherapy). Neo-adjuvant" chemotherapy should not be confused with curative chemotherapy, as the next procedure may "make up" for the failure of medical treatment.

• Neoadjuvant chemotherapy :

Its aim is to reduce the primary tumour and, if possible, facilitate removal surgery. For example, neo-adjuvant chemotherapy of the breast may make it possible to carry out valid conservative surgery and avoid the psychological trauma of mastectomy.

- Palliative chemotherapy :

Their aim is to prolong patient survival or improve comfort. In such cases, a cautious attitude is called for in the choice of combination therapy, which must be as non-toxic as possible and affordable.

3.3. ANTI-CANCER DRUGS

3.3.1.Definition (16):

An anti-cancer drug is designed to fight cancer by whatever mechanism. They can destroy malignant cells whose spontaneous growth knows no limits, or stop this growth, or help the body to get rid of them more effectively.

3.3.2.Classification (17) :

Anti-cancer drugs are classified by the WHO as antineoplastics and immunomodulators. Their target is the tumour cell, the accessibility of which varies in time and space according to its position in the cell cycle and its location in the body. A distinction can be made between "conventional" cancer chemotherapies, which act on cell proliferation (Table I), and targeted therapies whose activity is more specific to certain stages of oncogenesis (transduction of proliferation signals, cell death, angiogenesis, etc.). Their toxicity is generally lower than that of conventional therapies.

Table I: Classification of antiproliferative anti-cancer drugs according to their mechanisms of action.

Alkylants	
Formation of covalent adducts with DNA: inhibition of its transcription and synthesis. replication	
Nitrogen mustards	Cyclophosphamide, ifosfamide, chlorambucil, melphalan
Aziridines	Mitomycin
Platinum salts	Cisplatin, carboplatin, oxaliplatin
Nitrosoureas	Carmustine, folemustine, streptozocin
Intercalants	
Insertion between two consecutive DNA base pairs: inhibition of its transcription and its replication	
Anthracyclines doxorubicin, daunorubicin, epirubicin,	
Topoisomerase inhibitors	
Stabilisation of DNA cleavage complexes induced by topoisomerases: death cellular	
Camptothecins	Irinotecan, topotecan
Epipodophyllotoxins	Etoposide
Antimetabolites	
Structural analogues of compounds essential for nucleic acid synthesis	
Folinic acid antagonists Purine base analogues of bases pyrimidines	methotrexate, raltitrexed, pemetrexed 6-mercaptopurine, 6-thioguanine, fludarabine 5-fluorouracil, cytarabine, gemcitabine, azacytidine
MITOTIC SPINDLE POISONS	
Inhibition of the formation of the chromatic spindle that separates chromosomes during mitosis	
Vinca alkaloids Taxanes	Vinblastine, vincristine, vindesine, vinorelbine Paclitaxel, docetaxel, cabazitaxel

Immunomodulators (24) :

CTLA-4 inhibitors (Ipilimumab), PD-1 inhibitors (Pembrolizumab) and PD-L1 ligand inhibitors (Nivolumab and Atezolizumab) are all monoclonal antibodies that lift inhibition on T lymphocytes by preventing ligand-receptor interaction. They are known as immune checkpoint inhibitors. The result is activation of the lymphocytes, which attack the tumour cells, hence their therapeutic effect. The immunomodulators in the IMiD family, thalidomide and its derivatives lenalidomide and pomalidomide, have anti-angiogenic effects, a direct anti-tumour effect, interaction with the bone marrow microenvironment and immunomodulatory action. Interferon alpha 2A, alpha 2B and interleukin 2: these recombinant proteins have the same mechanisms of action and properties as their natural counterparts. They play an important immunostimulatory role in the expansion and activation of T lymphocytes.

Table II: Classification of immunomodulators used in cancer treatment

CTLA-4 inhibitors	Ipilimumab
PD-1 inhibitors	Pembrolizumab
PD-L1 ligand inhibitors	Nivolumab, Atezolizumab
IMiD	Thalidimide, Lenalidomide
Interferons and interleukins	Interferon Alpha 2A, Interleukin 2

3.3.3.Principle of associations (7):

In exceptional cases, a single drug is used; more often, a combination of 2 to 4 drugs is used, the action of which must be focused on tumour tissues and, on the contrary, diversified on normal tissues. The drugs used to treat a tumour must therefore be :

✓ All are active on the tumour in question;

✓ As different in toxicity as possible

✓ Different families and modes of action to reach as many cancer cells as possible, whatever their metabolic situation in relation to the cell cycle.

This is known as a therapeutic protocol. Chemotherapy protocols are determined according to the characteristics of the patient and his or her cancer. They alternate between phases in which the drugs are administered (the courses of treatment) and phases of rest to allow the body to recover. The choice of chemotherapy is based on a number of criteria: type of cancer and stage of progression, tumour location, age, state of health, medical history, etc. All these factors are taken into account by the medical team when proposing a personalised care programme (PPS) to the patient (25).

The number of courses of treatment also depends on the protocol, as does the rest interval between each administration of medication, which can range from 1 to 4 weeks. What's more, the treatment may change during the course of treatment (spacing out the courses of treatment, changing the molecules, etc.) in the light of its effectiveness and/or changes in the patient's state of health. During the first course of chemotherapy, a short period of in-patient monitoring is sometimes necessary, to check for possible reactions to the products. More than 70% of subsequent courses of chemotherapy are now administered on an outpatient basis: patients come to the hospital or clinic to receive their chemotherapy treatment, and then go home the same day. Hospitalisation at home is also possible in certain situations. Administration is then carried out by a specialist nurse, physiotherapist or dietician, depending on the case.

3.3.4.The main anti-cancer drugs and their mechanism of action (7): The majority of chemotherapy drugs can be subdivided into :

- Spindle/antimitotic poisons
- Alkylating agents
- Antimetabolites
- Anti-tumour antibiotics
- Topoisomerase inhibitors

All these drugs affect mitosis or DNA synthesis and function to some degree.

- Drugs acting on the spindle / antimitotic (21)

✓ Vinca-alkaloids (Vincristine, Vinblastine, Vindesine, Vinorelbine)

These are hemi-synthetic derivatives of a molecule extracted from the Madagascar periwinkle (Catharanthus roseus). They inhibit the polymerisation of tubulin, which plays an essential role in the formation of the mitotic spindle. They are the only true "antimitotics" and are used strictly intravenously; extravasation causes skin necrosis. Main indications: lymphoid leukaemia, lymphoma, Hodgkin's disease, non-small cell lung cancer, breast cancer.

✓ Taxanes (Paclitaxel, Docetaxel)

These are molecules extracted from yew (Taxus brevifolia Taxus baccata). They prevent tubulin polymerisation. They are also true antimitotics, blocking the cell in metaphase. They are administered strictly intravenously.

- Alkylating agents

These products are likely to induce an alkyl group on the DNA, forming stable bridges between the DNA chains that can no longer separate and play their role in mitosis. These drugs therefore act by altering the molecular structure of DNA. This group includes :

✓ Nitrogen mustards

These are : Chlorambucil, Cyclophosphamide, Ifosfamide and Melphalan. These are synthetic molecules (extracted from Saccharomyces cultures). These drugs form electrophilic molecules that bind covalently to DNA bases. These rearrangements cause DNA breaks and intra- or inter-strand bridges that inhibit the progress of DNA polymerase.

✓ Nitrosoureas

These are: endamusstin, carmutin, fotemustin, lomustin, streptozocin.

✓ Platinum salts

Cisplatin, Carboplatin, Oxaliplatin, Dacarbazine. These are synthetic molecules. They form electrophilic intermediates that bind covalently with nucleic bases and create intrastrand bridges that disrupt DNA replication.

- Structural analogues or antimetabolites (21)

They are antagonists of the purine and pyrimidine bases involved in nucleic acid synthesis.

✓ Purine analogues: mercaptopurine, clofaratine, cladribine.

✓ Pyrimidine analogues: Cytarabine, fluorouracil, capecitabine.

✓ Folic acid analogues: methotrexate, raltitrexed.

These drugs interfere with DNA synthesis by inhibiting the enzymes needed to make nucleotides. Methotrexate is a powerful folic acid antagonist.

- Anti-tumour antibiotics (21)

✓ Intercalating anthracyclines

These are intercalating antibiotics extracted from cultures of microscopic fungi (Streptomyces pencetius caesius) and chemically modified by hemi-synthesis. They are essentially doxorubicin and daunorubicin.

✓ Streptomyces

These are: actinomycin, bleomycin and mitomycin, which inhibit DNA transcription.

in RNA.

- Topoisomerase inhibitors :

Essential DNA repair enzymes (Excessive torsion)

- Topoisomerase I inhibitors

Topoisomerase I inhibitors are a recent class of anti-cancer drugs. They are water-soluble derivatives of Camptothecin, extracted from the Chinese plant Camptotheca acuminata: Irinotecan, Topotecan.

- Topoisomerase II inhibitors

They are derived from podopylla (podophyllum peltatum): podophylotoxin, etoposide, tenoposide.

3.3.5. Monographic study of some molecules:

3.3.5.1. Carboplatin :

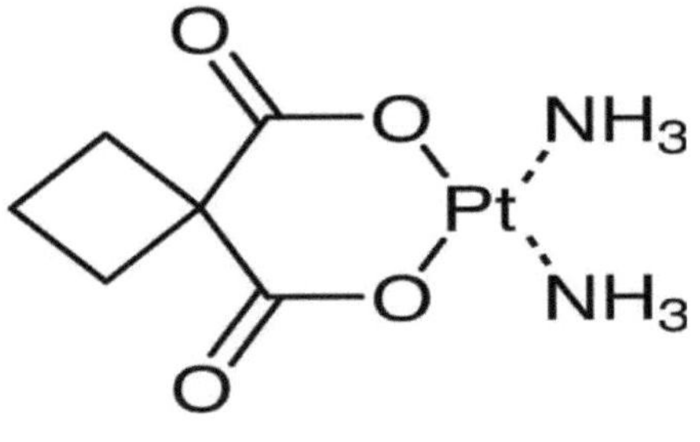

Figure 1: Chemical structure of carboplatin (18)

• Properties :

A platinum-derived alkylating agent that inhibits DNA synthesis by forming inter- and intracatenal bridges, with less toxicity at renal, auditory, neurological and digestive levels. It does not require hyperhydration or forced diuresis, but has more marked myelotoxicity (19).

• Indications (20):

✓ Small-cell bronchopulmonary cancer

✓ Ovarian cancer

✓ ENT cancer

• Contraindication (20):

✓ Breastfeeding

✓ Bone marrow aplasia

✓ Pregnancy

✓ Hypersensitivity to one of the ingredients

✓ Hypersensitivity to platinum derivatives

✓ Severe renal insufficiency: creatinine clearance

✓ Haemorrhagic tumour

3.3.5.2. Doxorubicin :

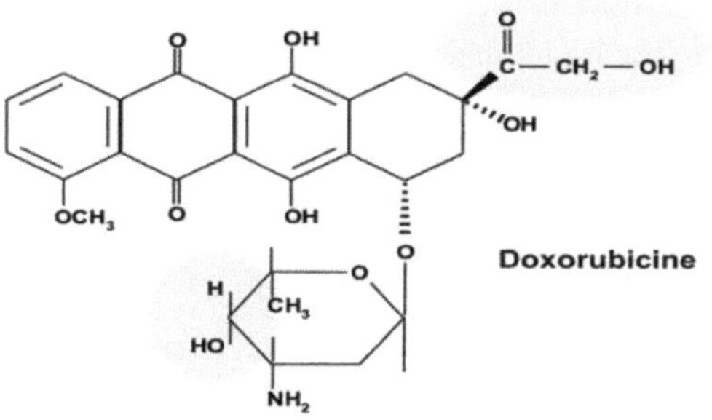

Figure 2: structure of doxorubicin (21)

• Mechanism of action (22):

Doxorubicin is a cytotoxic anthracycline antibiotic that may exert its anticancer effects by several mechanisms, including inhibition of topoisomerase II, intercalation with DNA and RNA polymerases, inhibition of helicase and formation of free radicals.

• Indications (21) :

There are quite a few of them;

- ✓ Breast carcinoma
- ✓ Bone and soft tissue sarcomas.
- ✓ Hodgkin's disease, non-Hodgkin's lymphoma
- ✓ Solid tumours in children
- ✓ Lung cancers
- ✓ Acute and chronic leukaemia

• Dosage (21) :

The usual dose is around 30 to 50 mg/m^2 every three weeks.

It is administered strictly by IV.

• Contraindications (23) :

- ✓ Breastfeeding
- ✓ Recent history of myocardial infarction
- ✓ Bone marrow aplasia
- ✓ Severe arrhythmia
- ✓ Maximum cumulative doses reached during previous anthracycline treatment
- ✓ Pregnancy
- ✓ Haematuria
- ✓ Hypersensitivity to one of the ingredients

✓ Hypersensitivity to anthracyclines

✓ Urinary tract infection

✓ Bladder inflammation

✓ Severe heart failure

✓ Severe liver failure

3.3.5.3. Paclitaxel :

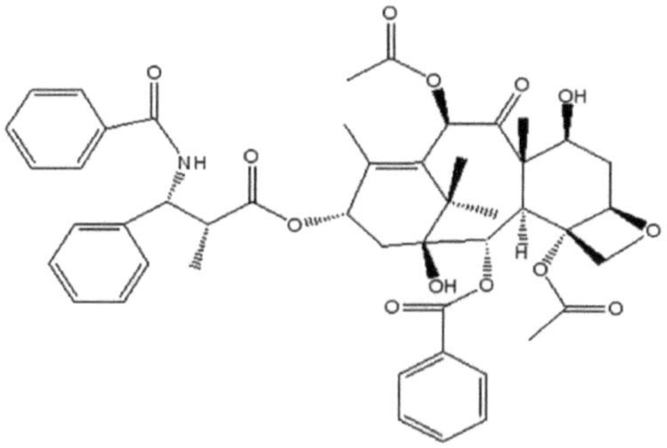

Figure 3: structure of paclitaxel (24)

• Mechanism of action (24) :

Unlike other tubulin-binding anti-cancer drugs, which prevent the assembly of tubulin into microtubules, paclitaxel promotes tubulin assembly. in microtubules and prevents microtubule dissociation, blocking cell cycle progression, preventing mitosis and inhibiting cancer cell growth.

Indications (25) :

✓ Non-small cell lung cancer

✓ Advanced ovarian cancer

✓ Metastatic ovarian cancer, 2nd-line treatment

✓ Breast cancer, adjuvant treatment

✓ Locally advanced breast cancer

- ✓ Metastatic breast cancer
- ✓ HER2 positive metastatic breast cancer
- ✓ AIDS-associated Kaposi's sarcoma, 2nd-line treatment

- Methods of administration (25) :

- ✓ Intravenous (infusion)
- ✓ To be diluted before administration
- ✓ Pre-medication with H1 and H2 antihistamines and corticosteroids
- ✓ Dosage to be adapted according to tolerance
- ✓ Treatment to be administered by course of treatment

- Contraindications (25) :

- ✓ Breastfeeding
- ✓ Pregnancy
- ✓ Hypersensitivity to one of the ingredients
- ✓ Uncontrolled infection
- ✓ Severe infection
- ✓ Severe liver failure
- ✓ Neutropenia.

METHODOLOGY

4.1. Study framework

The study was carried out at the M'PEWO private pharmacy, located in Lafiabougou (Rue 466 Porte 991) near the commune IV district hospital, which began operating on 01 September 1994. It has around forty staff (the head pharmacist, assistant pharmacists, interns, sales staff, trainees, assistants and security guards). It is open 24 hours a day, 7 days a week and can be contacted at 20293062. It is made up of :

- ✓ The office of the Pharmacist ;
- ✓ The assistants' office ;
- ✓ A sales area with 9 sales computers and a computer for the cash desk;
- ✓ Six product storage warehouses;
- ✓ A reception room for products ;
- ✓ A cloakroom, a dining room, toilets and a prayer area.

Dispensing was carried out by three (3) shifts, namely the morning shift, the evening shift and the on-call shift, with working hours of 8am to 4pm, 3pm to 10.30pm and 10pm to 8am respectively. During the survey period, patients with a prescription containing an anticancer drug were directed to the investigator, who dispensed the drug and took the opportunity to record the survey in the form of a questionnaire.

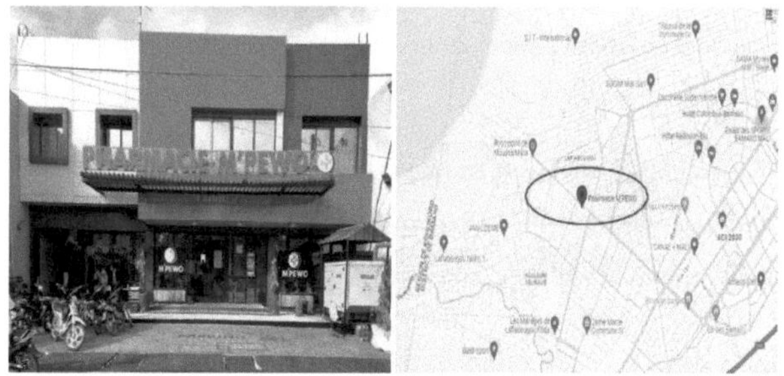

Figure 4: Photo and screenshot of the geolocation of the M'PEWO pharmacy (Photos Maiga).

4.2. Study period

Our study was carried out from 1 August 2023 to 18 July 2024 with a survey period of 6months from 1er December 2023 to 31 May 2024.

4.3. Type of study

This was a cross-sectional study.

4.4. Study population

The study population consisted of all prescriptions containing at least one anticancer drug.

4.5. Sampling

❖ Sampling technique :

We sampled all prescriptions meeting our inclusion criteria according to their order of arrival.

❖ Minimum sample size

It was calculated using the Daniel Schwartz formula:

$n = z^2 \times p(1 - p) / m^2$

n = sample size

z = confidence level according to the reduced centred normal distribution (for a confidence level of 95%, z = 1.96)

p = proportion of anticancer drugs available in a previous study. According to a study carried out in 2006, the proportion of anticancer drugs available in private pharmacies in Bamako was 25.78% (8).

m = Accuracy (for example, we want to know the real proportion to within 10%) n=1.962x 0.2578(1-0.2578)/0.01=73.50

After calculation, the minimum sample size is estimated at 74 prescriptions.

4.6. Inclusion criteria

Our study included : All prescriptions dispensed at the M'PEWO private pharmacy containing at least one anti-cancer drug whose holder agrees to be included in the study by providing additional information about the patient.

4.7. Non-inclusion criteria

Not included in our study:

- Any prescription that does not contain information about the prescriber;
- Anyone with a prescription for an anti-cancer drug in a hurry to leave the pharmacy, for whatever reason.

4.8. Data collection tools and techniques

Data were collected using a pre-established survey form. Patient data that did not appear on the prescription were requested from the holder by means of a face-to-face interview.

❖ Variables collected and operational definitions

• Socio-demographic characteristics of patients :
Age, gender, occupation, marital status.

• Type of cancer
Organ affected by the disease.

• Regulatory aspect of the order
The aim was to analyse whether the prescriptions complied with the rules of good prescribing. To do this, we analysed the following variables: information relating to the prescriber (qualification, telephone contact, stamp and signature), date on the prescription, information relating to the patient (first name and surname, age, sex), legibility of the prescription.

✓ Prescriptions (26): Prescribing is a medical act in its own right, based on a prescription. It involves prescribing something to a patient with the aim of curing an illness or pathology. It is governed by the Social Security Code, the Public Health Code and the Code of Medical Ethics.

✓ Prescription: any medium containing an anti-cancer drug, strictly presenting information on the prescriber (first name and surname or his stamp, signature or telephone contact). Information on the patient is requested; if it is not available, it is requested from the patient or the person accompanying the patient.

✓ The prescriber: This is the doctor (or other authorised person) who writes the prescription. They are identified by their stamp, which normally contains their first and last names, their qualifications and their contact details.

✓ Dispensing: Dispensing medicines to the patient is an act for which the pharmacist is directly responsible. It is a key activity in the management of a patient's medication and in ensuring its safety (27). It corresponds to an intellectual process including: pharmaceutical analysis of the prescription, where this exists, pharmaceutical analysis of a request in the absence of a prescription, monitoring and possible re-evaluation of the treatment, pharmaceutical advice, contribution to vigilance and handling of health alerts (28).

✓ Dispensers :

▪ Pharmacist: holder of a doctorate in pharmacy, working in the pharmacy as a pharmacist (full pharmacist and assistants).

▪ Intern: a student who has completed the 5th year of pharmacy and is training to work in a pharmacy with pharmacists.

▪ Trainee: any student from the 1ère to the 5è Année Pharmacie, following their training by working in the pharmacy with pharmacists.

▪ Vendor: any person with an employment contract who works in the pharmacy and has not completed pharmacist training.

✓ Determining the availability of anti-cancer drugs :

The anti-cancer drug prescribed is available in the pharmacy at the time of the request and in sufficient quantity, or the anti-cancer drug is not available or is in insufficient quantity.

• Identification of anti-cancer molecules :

The international non-proprietary name of the compound, the pharmaceutical form, the quantity requested and dispensed.

• Determining the average price of cancer drugs :

The total price of the anti-cancer molecules in each prescription was taken in order to determine the average price. The total price per prescription was divided into 8 bands with a range of 25,000 FCFA.

4.9. Data capture and analysis

Once the data had been collected, a search was made for missing data and outliers were corrected. SPSS® version 20 and Excel® were used for data entry and analysis. Categorical variables were presented as headcounts and percentages. The mean ± standard deviation or median and its range were calculated from the quantitative variables. Age was recoded into 6 age groups with an interval of 15 years. Price was recoded into 8 bands with a 25,000FCFA interval. The information was presented in the form of tables and graphs.

4.10. Ethical and deontological considerations

The survey in the pharmacy was authorised by the pharmacist in charge of the M'PEWO pharmacy before it was carried out. The study was conducted in accordance with the ethical principles of medical research, in particular the obtaining of free and informed verbal consent from patients or accompanying persons before including them in the study, and the preservation of data confidentiality. The survey forms were anonymous. We did not record any personal information about the patients who owned the prescriptions or about the prescriber. The identification of the patient by people outside our study was avoided; only the number of the forms was used to identify the data. The information retained on our survey form was that which was essential for our study.

RESULTS

A total of 102 prescriptions from 85 patients were analysed.

5.1. Breakdown of cancer patients by socio-demographic characteristics

5.1.1.Breakdown by gender

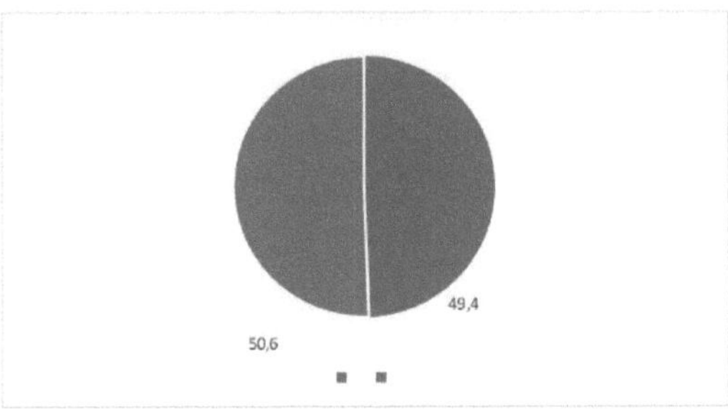

Figure 5: Gender distribution of cancer patients based on prescriptions received at the M'PEWO pharmacy from December 2023 to May 2024, n=85.

Females accounted for 50.6% of our sample. The sex ratio was 0.98.

5.1.2.Breakdown by age

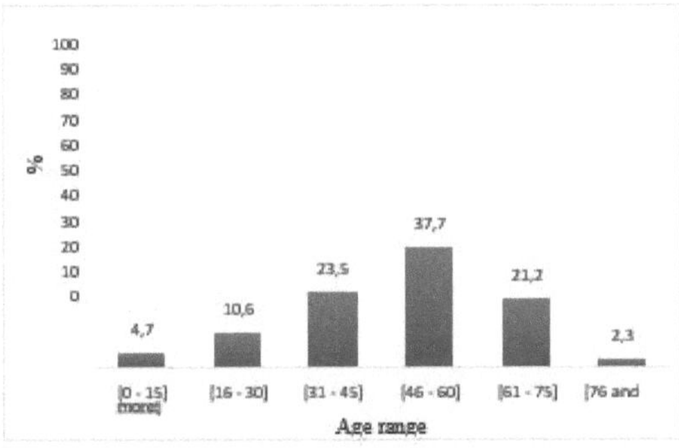

Figure 6: Breakdown of cancer patients by age, based on prescriptions received at the M'PEWO pharmacy from December 2023 to May 2024, n=85.

The [46 - 60] age group accounted for 37.7% (n=32).

The mean age was 48.86 ± 16.45 years.

5.1.3.Breakdown of patients by profession

Table III: Occupational distribution of cancer patients based on prescriptions received at the M'PEWO pharmacy from December 2023 to May 2024, n=85.

Profession	n	%
Agro-pastoral	9	10,6
Unemployment	5	5,9
Retailer	14	16,5
Student	4	4,7
Civil servant	10	11,8
Engineer	3	3,5
Housekeeper	27	31,8
Military	2	2,3
Worker	9	10,6
Retirement	2	2,3
Total	85	100,0

Housekeeping accounted for 31.8%.

Study of the dispensing of anti-cancer drugs in private pharmacies

M'PEWO from August 2023 to July 2024

5.1.4.Breakdown by marital status

Table IV: Distribution according to marital status of cancer patients based on prescriptions received at the M'PEWO pharmacy from December 2023 to May 2024, n=85.

Marital status of patients	n	%
Married	62	72,9
Single	10	11,8
Divorced	2	2,4
Widow(er)	11	12,9
Total	85	100,0
Marital status Married represented 72.9%.		

5.2. Breakdown by type of cancer :

Table V: Breakdown of cancer patients by type of cancer from prescriptions received at the M'PEWO pharmacy from December 2023 to May 2024, n=85.

Type of cancer n	%	
Spleen cancer 1	1,2	
Bladder cancer 5	5,9	
Lung cancer 5	5,9	
Breast cancer 12	14,1	
Prostate cancer 2	2,3	
Eye cancer 2	2,3	
Skin cancers 9	10,6	
Digestive cancers 29	34,1	
Gynaecological cancers 14	16,5	
Haematological cancers 2	2,3	
Metastasis 4	4,8	
Total 85	100,0	
*Digestive cancers: oesophageal cancer 8.2%; gastrointestinal cancer 8.2%.	stomach cancer (14.1%)	from

colon/rectum 10.6%; liver cancer 1.2%.

**Gynaecological cancers: cervical cancer 10.6%; ovarian cancer 5.9%.

***Haematological cancers: blood cancer 1.2%; AML 1.2%. Digestive cancers accounted for 34.1% of our sample.

Breast cancer and stomach cancer each accounted for 14.1%.

5.3. Identifying the regulatory characteristics of prescriptions

5.3.1. Breakdown by prescriber qualification

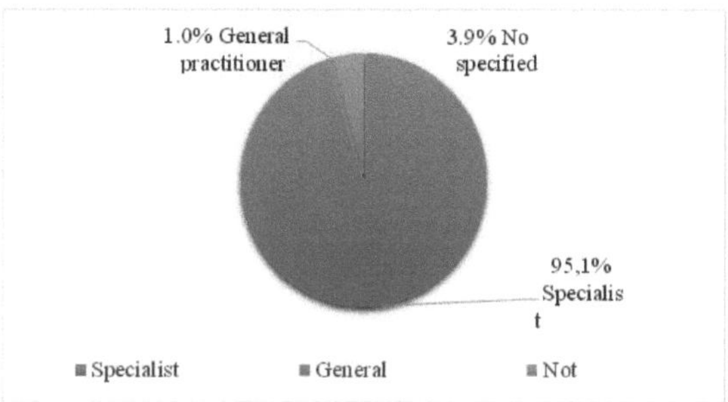

Figure 7: Distribution according to prescriber qualification of cancer patients from prescriptions received at the M'PEWO pharmacy from December 2023 to May 2024, n=102.

Specialist doctors were the prescribers (95.1%).

5.3.2.Breakdown by provider status

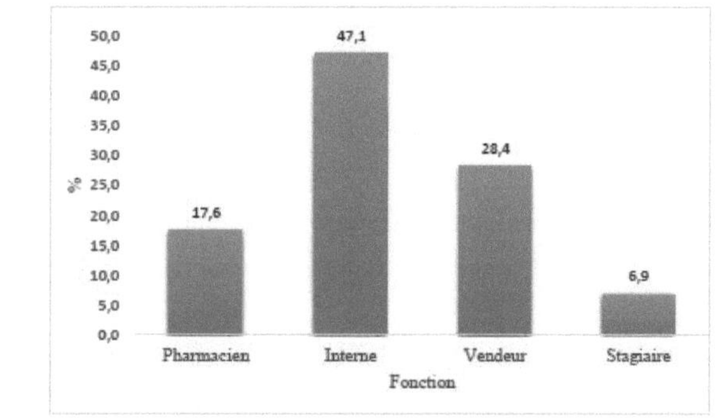

Figure 8: Distribution according to dispensing status of cancer patients from prescriptions received at the M'PEWO pharmacy from December 2023 to May 2024, n=102.

47.1% of prescriptions were filled by interns.

5.3.3.Practitioner's signature and stamp on prescription

Table VI: Distribution according to signature and practitioner's stamp on the prescription of cancer patients seen at the M'PEWO pharmacy from December 2023 to May 2024, n=102.

Practitioner's signature and stamp on prescription	n	%
Presence	97	95,1
Absence	5	4,9
Total	102	100,0

Sealed prescriptions accounted for 95.1% of our sample.

5.3.4.Distribution according to the presence of the date on the prescription

Table VII: Distribution according to the date on the prescription of cancer patients received at the M'PEWO pharmacy from December 2023 to May 2024, n=102

Order	n	%
Dated	87	85,3
Undated	15	14,7
Total	102	100,0

Dated prescriptions accounted for 85.3% of our sample.

5.3.5. Telephone contact for the prescriber on the prescription

Table VIII: Distribution according to telephone contact on the prescription of cancer patients seen at the M'PEWO pharmacy from December 2023 to May 2024, n=102.

Telephone contact about the prescription	n	%
Telephone contact	98	96,1
No telephone contact	4	3,9
Total	102	100,0

Telephone contact with the prescriber was present on 96.1% of prescriptions.

5.3.6. Presence of patient information and legibility of prescriptions

Table IX: Distribution according to the presence of patient information and the legibility of the prescription of cancer patients seen at the M'PEWO pharmacy from December 2023 to May 2024, n=102.

Order	n	%
Presence of patient information	102	100,0
Failure to provide patient information	0	0,0
Total	102	100,0
Readable	102	100,0
Not readable	0	0,0
Total	102	100,0

The prescriptions contained patient information and were 100% legible.

5.4. Availability of cancer drugs

5.4.1.Breakdown by availability of anti-cancer drugs

Table X: Distribution according to availability of anticancer drugs of cancer patients based on prescriptions received at the M'PEWO pharmacy from December 2023 to May 2024, n=102.

Anti-cancer drug prescribed	n	%
Available at	101	99,0
Break	1	1,0
Total	102	100,0

99% of anti-cancer drugs were available during our survey. Only one molecule was unavailable on a prescription, representing 1%.

5.4.2.Breakdown by number of anticancer drugs prescribed

Table XI: Distribution according to the number of anticancer drugs on the prescription of cancer patients seen at the M'PEWO pharmacy from December 2023 to May 2024, n=102.

Number of anti-cancer drugs on prescription	n	%
1	42	41,2
2	34	33,3
3	21	20,6
4	5	4,9
Total	102	100,0

Prescriptions for a single anti-cancer drug accounted for 41.2%.

5.5. Identification of anti-cancer molecules

5.5.1.Breakdown of cancer drugs by pharmaceutical form

Table XII: Breakdown by pharmaceutical form of anticancer drugs for cancer patients based on prescriptions received at the M'PEWO pharmacy from December 2023 to May 2024, n=102.

Pharmaceutical form	n	%
Injectable	94	92,2
Tablet	8	7,8
Total	102	100,0

The injectable form accounted for 92.2% of our sample.

The 5.5.2. Breakdown of anticancer drugs by total number dispensed

Table XIII: Distribution according to the total number of anti-cancer drugs dispensed to cancer patients based on prescriptions received at the M'PEWO pharmacy from December 2023 to May 2024 (n=192 molecules)

Cytotoxic molecules	n	%
Vinca-alkaloids	3	1,6
Taxanes	33	17,2
Nitrogen mustards	8	4,2
Platinum salts	53	27,6
Antimetabolites	78	40,6
Intercalating anthracyclines	9	4,7
Topoisomerase inhibitors	6	3,1
Protein kinase inhibitors	2	1
Total	192	100

*Vinca-alkaloids: Vincritine 1.6%.

**Taxanes: Paclitaxel 13%; Docetaxel 4.2%.

***Nitrogen mustards: Cyclophosphamide 3.7%; Mephalan 0.5%.

**** Platinum salts: Carboplatin 15.6%; Oxaliplatin 2.1%; Cisplatin 9.9%.

****** Antimetabolites: Folinic acid 15.1%; Capecitabine 2.6%; Cytarabine 0.5%; Fluoro uracil 14.6%; Gemcitabine 5.2%; Methotrexate 1%; Zoledronic acid 3%.

******Intercalating anthracyclines: Doxorubicin 4.7%.

*******Topoisomerase inhibitors: Etoposide 0.5%; Irinotecan 2.6%.

******** Protein kinase inhibitors: Sorafenib 1%. Antimetabolites accounted for 40.6% of our sample. Carboplatin accounted for 15.6% of our sample.

5.6. Determining the average price of anti-cancer drugs

5.6.1. Breakdown of prescriptions by total price of anti-cancer drugs

Table XIV: Breakdown by total prescription price of cancer patients seen at the M'PEWO pharmacy from December 2023 to May 2024, n=102.

Total price range in CFA francs per prescription	n	%
14000 à 39000	26	25,5
39001 à 64000	30	29,4
64001 à 89000	18	17,7
89001 à 114000	13	12,7
114001 à 139000	7	6,9
139001 à 164000	2	2,0
164001 à 189000	3	2,9
189001 and more	3	2,9
Total	102	100,0

The price range 39001 to 64000 was represented by 29.4% of our sample. The average price was 74285.05 FCFA ±58766.028 FCFA...

5.6.2.Breakdown of prescriptions according to the presence or absence of adjuvant drugs

Table XV: Distribution according to the presence or absence of adjuvant molecules of cancer patients based on prescriptions received at the M'PEWO pharmacy from December 2023 to May 2024, n=102.

Order	n	%
With additive	35	34,3
No additives	67	65,7
Total	102	100,0

Prescriptions without adjuvant molecules accounted for 66% of our sample.

5.6.3.Breakdown by total number of adjuvant drugs dispensed

Table XVI: Distribution according to the total number dispensed of adjuvant molecules for cancer patients based on prescriptions received at the M'PEWO pharmacy from December 2023 to May 2024, (n=72 molecules).

Adjuvant molecule	n	%
Dexamethasone	15	20,8
Levosulpiride and similar products	12	16,7
Loperamide	6	8,3
Morphine and derivatives	2	2,8
Omeprazole and other PPIs	14	19,5
Ondansetron	15	20,8
Prednisone and Methylprednisone	8	11,1
Total	72	100

Of a total of 72 adjuvant drugs dispensed, dexamethasone and ondansetron were the most commonly used. prescribed to 20.8% of our sample each.

COMMENTS AND DISCUSSION

This was a cross-sectional study with a prospective survey of 6 months (1er December 2023 to 31 May 2024) for 102 prescriptions belonging to 85 patients. This study focused on patients or those accompanying patients who came to the M'PEWO pharmacy with at least one prescription from an oncology department and containing at least one anti-cancer molecule.

6.1. **Limitations and difficulties encountered**

The fact that patients were not present in the pharmacy meant that certain socio-demographic data such as weight, height and body mass index (BMI) were not taken into account. This could constitute an information bias. There are few similar studies in Mali to compare results.

6.2. Socio-demographic characteristics

- Gender

We found that women predominated, accounting for just over half of our sample. **Sidibé F in 2023**, on Contribution à l'amélioration de la dispensation des médicaments anticancéreux au CHU du Point G, obtained 69.4% for women (7) and **Kamaté K in 2007,** on the Problématique de l'Accès Aux Médicaments Anticancéreux Au Mali, reported 70.96% for women (29). This result could be explained by the cancer rate, which is higher in women than in men in Mali (30).

- Age

The [46-60] age group was the most represented, followed by the [31-45] age group in our sample. **Ly M in 2001,** on the Itinerary of cancer patients seen in the haematology-oncology and internal medicine departments of Point G Hospital, found that the [46-60] and [31-45] age groups were the most frequent with 29.7% and 23.6% respectively (31). **Fofana M in 2022**, on Analyse de la prescription et la dispensation des anticancéreux au mali : cas de l'hôpital du mali (32), found the age groups [41-50] and [51-60] to be the most prevalent with 28.7% and 24.7% respectively. This could be explained by the youth of the Malian population, whose total life expectancy is 62.8 years (33).

- **Profession**

We found that over a quarter of our patients were housewives. Shopkeepers came 2nd. Our results are similar to those of **Majio RP in 2022**, on the Evaluation of palliative care needs in the haematology and medical oncology department of the CHU Point G (34), which found that housewives were in the majority, followed by shopkeepers. The prevalence of housewives could be explained by the prevalence of women.

- **Marital status**

Married people represented almost three quarters of our sample. This predominance was also reported by **Kamaté K in 2007**, who obtained 64.52% of married patients (29), by **Koné FT in 2019** who reported 77% of married patients (35). In 2022**, Wembe SDM**, in his study on the epidemiological and clinical profile of patients in the palliative and supportive care unit at the CHU Point G, obtained 81.71% of married patients (36). This result could be linked to the predominance of housewives, which is the main function of housewives in Mali.

6.3. **Type of cancer**

Digestive cancers accounted for almost a third of the sample. Breast and stomach cancer were the most common. **Sidibe F in 2023,** reported in his study a predominance of breast cancer(7). This higher rate of breast and stomach cancer could be explained by the lack of prevention and late diagnosis.

6.4. **Regulatory aspect of the orders**

Almost all the prescriptions were written by medical specialists. They were all legible, and most were sealed and dated. The prescriber's telephone contact was present on almost all of them. In Mali, cancer treatment is a specialised field. In most cases, general practitioners refer patients to specialists for treatment.

6.5. **Availability of cancer drugs**

Anticancer molecules were 99% available during our survey. This good availability could explain the involvement of the M'PEWO pharmacy in the management of its stock.

- Total number of anticancer drugs prescribed per prescription

Prescriptions containing a single anti-cancer drug were the most common, accounting for around half of our sample. This result could b e explained by the fact that anti-cancer drugs in public hospitals, where when they were unavailable patients sought the

anti-cancer molecule unavailable in private pharmacies.

- The pharmaceutical form of anti-cancer drugs

Almost all the anticancer drugs dispensed during our study were injectables. This result could be explained by the delay in diagnosis, as oral treatment was no longer an option.

6.6. Anti-cancer molecules used

- Total number of anti-cancer drugs dispensed

Carboplatin was the most widely dispensed anticancer drug in our study (15.6%). This could be explained by the fact that it is free in hospitals and that it is very often out of stock in hospitals, hence its greater demand in private pharmacies.

6.7. **Total price of cancer drugs**

The price range [39001 - 64000] FCFA was the most represented in our sample with an average price of 74285 FCFA±58766.028. This may explain the high cost of the treatments offered and patients' complaints about the high cost of anticancer drugs, as emphasised by **Kamaté K** in his study (29).

CONCLUSION AND RECOMMENDATIONS

7.1. CONCLUSION

The study involved 102 registered prescriptions belonging to 85 patients. Women were more frequent. The [46-60] age group accounted for 37.7%. The mean age was 48.86 ± 16.45 years. Breast and gastric cancer were the most common cancers, each accounting for 14.1%. Almost all the prescriptions were written by specialist doctors. They were all legible, and most were sealed and dated. The availability of anti-cancer drugs was 99%. Carboplatin was the most dispensed anticancer drug, with 15.6%. The average price of the prescription was 74285 FCFA±58766.028 FCFA.A future study could be carried out in several pharmacies and focus on the following aspects economic aspects of dispensing, in particular the burden on the patient.

7.2. RECOMMENDATIONS

• At the M'PEWO pharmacy

Please ensure the availability of anti-cancer drugs;

Refer the patient directly to an oncologist if a tumour is suspected.

• Ministry of Health

Include anti-cancer drugs and other pharmaceutical products used in the treatment of cancer on the national list of essential medicines, and Involve insurance companies, especially the compulsory health insurance scheme (AMO), in paying for them.

• To the health and political authorities

Organise public awareness sessions on early cancer detection; train health workers in cancer treatment and create dedicated facilities and equipment.

• To patients and the general public:

Participate in screening campaigns for cancer and certain infectious diseases (AIDS, hepatitis, human papillomavirus);

Avoid as far as possible risk factors for cancer such as: tobacco, alcohol, a sedentary lifestyle, viral and bacterial infections, poor diet, exposure to UV rays and ionising radiation, etc.

REFERENCES

1. Ligue contre le cancer. Cancer, definition [Internet]. 2023 [cited 15 Jan 2024]. Available from: https://www.ligue-cancer.net/articles/le-cancer-definition

2. Mbalawa CG, Godet J, Gueye SM. cancers in francophone Africa [Internet]. La Ligue Nationale contre le Cancer (France); 2017 [cited 11 Jan 2024]. 135 p. Available from: https://www.iccp-portal.org/system/files/resources/LivreCancer.pdf

3. WHO (Regional Office for Africa). World Cancer Day 2022 [Internet]. 2023 [cited 28 Nov 2023]. Available from: https://www.afro.who.int/fr/regional- director/speeches-messages/world-cancer-day-2022

4. Ballo M, Guindo AA, Traoré M dit S, Touré M, Dao F, Traoré K, et al. Gratuité des Anticancéreux au Mali : Évaluation des Facteurs Limitant la Disponibilité des Anticancéreux au Centre Hospitalier Universitaire du Point G: Factors limiting the gratuity of anticancer drugs in Mali. Health Sci Dis. 2022;23(1):92-6.

5. Globocan. Mali fact sheets 2021 [Internet]. 2021. Available at: https://gco.iarc.fr/today/data/factsheets/populations/466-mali-fact-sheets.pdf

6. Jeune Afrique. JeuneAfrique.com. [cited 9 Nov 2023]. Health: 10 things to know about cancer in Africa - Jeune Afrique. Available at: https://www.jeuneafrique.com/33734/societe/sant-10-choses-savoir-sur-le-cancer-en-afrique/

7. Sidibé F. Contribution to improving the dispensing of medicines anticancer drugs at the CHU du Point G. USTTB.2023;N°003:83p;

8. Bah S, Bengaly L, Cisse BS, Coulibaly S, Dembele AK, Dembele M, et al. Factors limiting access to anticancer drugs in a Bamako University Hospital; Mali. Mali Méd En Ligne. 2011;37-40.

9. Wikipedia. Tumour. In 2023 [cited 30 Jan 2024]. Available from: https://fr.wikipedia.org/w/index.php?title=Tumeur&oldid=209207166

10. French National Cancer Institute. Types and stages of cancer - What is cancer? [Internet]. [cited 9 nov 2023]. Available from: https://www.e-cancer.fr/Comprendre- prevenir-depister/Qu-est-ce-qu'un-cancer/Types-et-stades-des-cancers

11. MSD manual. Development and spread of cancer - Cancer [Internet]. [cited 15 Jan 2024].

Available from: https://www.msdmanuals.com/fr/accueil/cancer/pr%C3%A9sentation-des-cancers/d%C3%A9development-and-spread-of-cancer

12. WHO. Cancer [Internet]. [cited 6 Nov 2023]. Available from: https://www.who.int/fr/news-room/fact-sheets/detail/cancer

13. Globocan. Mali Cancer Tomorrow [Internet]. [cited 17 Jan 2024]. Available from: https://gco.iarc.fr/tomorrow/en/dataviz/isotype?populations=466&single_unit=1000&group_populations=1&multiple_populations=1

14. JSTM JS et T du. Mali: 1,545 cases of cancer recorded in Bamako in 2019 | JSTM [Internet]. 2021 [cited 17 Jan 2024]. Available from: https://www.jstm.org/mali-1-545-cas-de-cancer-recenses-a-bamako-en-2019/

15. Ligue contre le cancer. Chemotherapy | Ligue contre le cancer [Internet]. [cited 21 Jan 2024]. Available from: https://www.ligue-cancer.net/les-traitements/la-chimiotherapie

16. Cazivassilio D. Anticancer drugs: treatment, definition [Internet]. [cited 10 Jul 2024]. Available at: https://www.docteurclic.com/traitement/medicaments-anticancereux.aspx

17. Kamissoko S. Sécurisation du circuit des cytotoxiques au Centre Hospitalier Universitaire Point G : de la prescription à la gestion des déchets. USTTB.2021;N°00:85p;

18. Zhang C, Xu C, Gao X, Yao Q. Platinum-based drugs for cancer therapy and anti-tumor strategies. Theranostics. 7 Feb 2022;12(5):2115-32.

19. Vital Durand D, Le Jeunne C. Guide pratique des médicaments [Internet]. Maloine. France; 2023. 1998 p. Available at: www.maloine.fr

20. VIDAL. Carboplatin: active substance with therapeutic effect [Internet]. [cited 10 Jul 2024]. Available at: https://www.vidal.fr/medicaments/substances/carboplatine-810.html

21. Roamba M. Evaluation de la préparation et de l'administration de la chimiothérapie à l'unité d'oncologie pédiatrique CHU Gabriel TOURE. USTTB.2020;N°00:97p;

22. NetCancer. Doxorubicin [Internet]. [cited 10 Jul 2024]. Available from: https://netcancer.net/medicament/adriamycine/

23. VIDAL. Doxorubicin: active substance with therapeutic effect [Internet]. [cited 10 Jul 2024]. Available at: https://www.vidal.fr/medicaments/substances/doxorubicine-6769.html

24. Zhu L, Chen L. Progress in research on paclitaxel and tumor immunotherapy. Cell Mol

Biol Lett. June 13, 2019;24(1):40.

25. Vidal. VIDAL. [cited 1 Feb 2024]. Paclitaxel: active substance with therapeutic effect. Available at: https://www.vidal.fr/medicaments/substances/paclitaxel-4403.html

26. PagesJaunes. PagesJaunes.fr. [cited 8 Jul 2024]. Prescription médicale - PagesJaunes. Available at: https://medicament.pagesjaunes.fr

27. WEKA. What is drug dispensing? [Internet]. [cited 9 nov 2023]. Available from: https://www.weka.fr/sante/dossier-pratique/maitrise-des-risques-et-de-la- qualite-dt86/qu-est-ce-que-la-dispensation-du-medicament-5322/

28. Collège des Pharmaciens. L'acte de dispensation - Guide de stage de pratique professionnelle en officine [Internet]. 2020 [cited 8 Jul 2024]. Available from: https://cpcms.fr/guide-stage/knowledge-base/lacte-de-dispensation/

29. Kamaté K. The problem of access to anti-cancer drugs in Mali. USTTB.2007;N°07P29:140p;

30. Ngassa Piotie P. Cancer incidence and mortality in Mali: data from the Mali Cancer Registry. cancer from 1995 to 2004. USTTB.2006;N°00:93p;

31. Ly M. Itinéraire des malades cancéreux vus dans les services d'hématologie-oncologie et de médecine interne de l'Hôpital du Point G. USTTB.2001;N°36:116p;

32. Fofana M. Analyse de la prescription et la dispensation des anticancéreux au Mali : Cas de l'Hôpital du Mali. USTTB.2022;N°00:88p;

33. World Life Expectancy. Life expectancy in Mali [Internet]. [cited 13 Jul 2024]. Available from: https://www.worldlifeexpectancy.com/fr/mali-life-expectancy

34. Majio RP. Evaluation of palliative care needs in the haematology and medical oncology department of CHU Point G. USTTB.2022;N°00:108p;

35. Koné FT. Evaluation of drug management of cancer pain in the medical oncology department of the CHU Luxembourg. USTTB.2019;N°00:101p;

36. WEMBE SDMC. Profil épidémio-clinique des patients en unité de soins palliatifs et soins de support du CHU Point G. USTTB.2022;N°00:84p;

37. Legifrance. Arrêté du 28 novembre 2016 relatif aux bonnes pratiques de dispensation des médicaments dans les pharmacies d'officine, les pharmacies mutualistes et les pharmacies de

secours minières, mentionnées à l'article L. 5121-5 du code de la santé publique - Légifrance [Internet]. [cited 13 Jul 2024]. Available from: https://www.legifrance.gouv.fr/jorf/id/JORFTEXT000033507633

APPENDICES

Survey form

N°...

I - PATIENT IDENTIFICATION

Dispensing date:

Age (in years):

Gender: □Male□Female

Marital status: □Married□Single□ Widowed □Divorced

Profession :organ affected or type of cancer

II - Information on molecules

Anti-cancer molecules

Molecule(s)	Shape pharmaceutical	Quantity(ies) requested(s)	Quantity(ies) dispensed

Has the patient had all the products prescribed□Yes□No

If not, the products on the prescription are out of stock:

Price total of cancer drugs from prescription (inFCFA) :

Associated molecules :

Molecule(s)	Shape pharmaceutical	Quantity(ies) requested(s)	Quantities dispensed

III- Dispensing information

Provider status

Pharmacist /............/Internal /............/ Salesman//Trainee/... /

IV- Information relating to the prescriber and regulatory aspects of the order :

1. Qualification of the prescriber

□ Specialist **doctor** □ Specialist doctor (DES) □ General practitioner

□Not specified

2. Telephone contact(s) of the prescriber :□Yes□No

3. Signature and stamp of prescriber :□Yes□No
4. Date on prescription:□ Yes□No
5. Patient information:□Yes□No
6. Legibility of the prescription : □ Yes□No

FACT SHEET

First name: Souleymane

Name: MAIGA

Country of origin: Mali

Nationality: Malian

E-mail address: souleymanemaiga9489@gmail.com

Contact: +223 94 89 69 44

Title of thesis: Study of the dispensing of anti-cancer drugs in pharmacies private M'PEWO from August 2023 to July 2024

Academic year: 2023-2024 **Date of defence**: 18/07/2024 **City of defence**: Bamako

Depository: Faculty of Pharmacy Library

Sector of interest: Public health.

SUMMARY

Introduction: An anti-cancer drug is intended to fight cancer, whatever its mechanism. It is designed to destroy or stop the growth of malignant cells or to help the body get rid of them more effectively. Dispensing is the pharmaceutical act which combines the dispensing of medicines, the pharmaceutical analysis of the medical prescription and the provision of information and advice necessary for the correct use of medicines (37).

Objective: To study the dispensing of anti-cancer drugs in private pharmacies M'PEWO from August 2023 to July 2024.

Method: This was a cross-sectional study with a 6-month survey period from 1er December 2023 to 31 May 2024.

Results: The study involved 102 registered prescriptions belonging to 85 patients. Women were more frequent. The [46-60] age group accounted for 37.7%. The mean age was 48.86 ± 16.45 years. Breast and gastric cancer were the most common cancers, each accounting for 14.1%. Almost all the prescriptions were written by specialist doctors. They were all legible, and most were sealed and dated. The availability of anti-cancer drugs was 99%. Carboplatin was the most dispensed anticancer drug, with 15.6%. The average price of the prescription was 74285 FCFA±58766.028 FCFA.

Conclusion : A future study could be carried out in several pharmacies, focusing on economic aspects of dispensing, in particular the burden on the patient.

Key words: Dispensing, anti-cancer drugs, private pharmacy.

PHARMACIST'S OATH

I swear, in the presence of the masters of the Faculty, the councillors of the order of pharmacists and of my fellow students:

To honour those who have instructed me in the precepts of my art and to show them my gratitude. recognition by remaining faithful to their teaching;

To practise my profession conscientiously, in the interests of public health, and to comply not only with current legislation, but also with the rules of honour, probity and disinterestedness.

Never to forget my responsibility and duties towards patients and their human dignity.

Under no circumstances will I agree to use my knowledge and status to corrupt the and encourage criminal acts.

May men esteem me if I am faithful to my promises. May I be shamed and despised by my colleagues if I fail to do so.

I SWEAR IT.

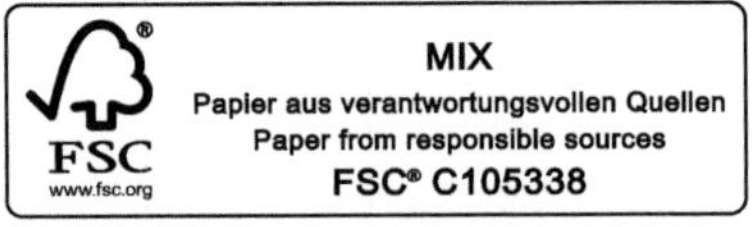

Printed by Books on Demand GmbH, Norderstedt / Germany